USING

S-ADENOSYL METHIONINE

FOR BEGINNERS

Essential Primer To Boost Your Health, Improve Joint Function, Optimal Well-Being, Liver Function, Impact On Mood And More

DR. SPARKS RUBIO

DISCLAIMER

The information presented in this book is intended for general informational purposes only. It is not a substitute for professional medical advice, diagnosis, or treatment.

The author and publisher of this book have made every effort to ensure that the information provided is accurate and up-to-date at the time of publication. However, medical and scientific knowledge is constantly evolving, and new research may emerge. Therefore, the information in this book should not be considered a definitive source for medical or nutritional advice.

It is essential to consult with a qualified healthcare professional before making any decisions.

The author and publisher disclaim any liability for any adverse outcomes or consequences resulting from the use or misuse of the information in this book. Readers are urged to use their discretion and judgment when making decisions about their health and wellness.

By reading this book, you agree to do so at your own risk and should not use it as a substitute for professional medical advice or treatment.

TABLE OF CONTENTS

CHAPTER ONE 8

  INTRODUCTION TO S-ADENOSYL METHIONINE 8

    WHAT IS SAME? 8

    SAME SYNOPSIS 9

    HISTORICAL BACKGROUND 11

CHAPTER TWO 14

  SAME IN HUMAN BODY 14

    THE PART SAME PLAYS.................................14

    BIOSYNTHESIS OF SAME 15

    METABOLISM SAME.....................................16

CHAPTER THREE 20

  THE ADVANTAGES OF SAME 20

    SAME FOR MENTAL AND MOOD DISORDERS 20

    DEPRESSION AND SAME 22

    SAME AND UNEASE.....................................23

    COGNITIVE FUNCTION AND SAME.....................24

CHAPTER FOUR 26

  SAME AND WELLNESS...................................26

    SAME FOR HEALTHY JOINTS...........................26

    SAME FOR HEPATIC FUNCTION 28

HEART HEALTH WITH SAME.................................30

CHAPTER FIVE 32

SAME AS AN ADD-ON 32

FORMS AND AMOUNTS 32

DISTINCT SAME FORMS 33

CHOOSING THE APPROPRIATE DOSAGE 34

SELECTING THE APPROPRIATE SAME...................35

ASPECTS TO THINK ABOUT 36

CHAPTER SIX 38

POSSIBLE ADVERSE REACTIONS AND CONCURRENT EVENTS...38

FREQUENT ADVERSE EVENTS..............................38

DRUG-DRUG RELATIONS................................40

CHAPTER SEVEN..44

PARTICULAR POPULATIONS AND SAME 44

SAME YOUNGSTERS 44

SAME FOR SENIOR CITIZENS 46

SAME THROUGHOUT HER PREGNANCY AND 48

CHAPTER EIGHT 50

INCLUDING SAME IN YOUR DAILY ACTIVITIES 50

DIET AND SAME 50

SOURCES OF SAME IN DIET 51

SAME AND DIETARY ASSISTANCE 52

CHAPTER NINE 56

SAME IN COMBINATION WITH OTHER SUPPLEMENTS
....56

COOPERATION WITH OTHER ELEMENTS 56

VITAMIN SUPPLEMENTS AND SAME....................57

SUGGESTIONS FOR SAME 58

TOP TECHNIQUES....................................60

OBSERVING AND MODIFYING.............................61

CHAPTER TEN 64

THE PROSPECTS FOR SAME STUDIES 64

CURRENT RESEARCH AND UPCOMING PROJECTS 64

RECENT RESEARCH 65

POTENTIAL APPLICATIONS....................................68

CHAPTER ELEVEN 72

CHALLENGES FACED.................................72

HEALTHCARE PROFESSIONALS' PERSPECTIVES 75

CHAPTER ONE

INTRODUCTION TO S-ADENOSYL METHIONINE

WHAT IS SAME?

SAMe, or S-Adenosyl methionine in scientific parlance, is a naturally occurring substance that is essential to many different metabolic activities in the body. Since its discovery by Giulio Cantoni in 1952, SAMe has attracted a lot of interest due to its possible health advantages, especially liver function, joint health, and mood management. It is noteworthy for its role in the methylation process, which is where it acts as a methyl donor to facilitate the creation of several molecules essential to the proper operation of the body. Due to its reported benefits for liver ailments, osteoarthritis, and mood disorders, SAMe has become more well-known as a dietary supplement and medicinal agent. This has piqued the curiosity of both the general public and the scientific community.

SAME SYNOPSIS

In the realm of mental health, SAMe has become a prominent actor. An increasing amount of studies indicates that SAMe may have natural antidepressant properties. It is thought to aid in the manufacture of neurotransmitters that are vital for controlling mood and mental health, including serotonin and dopamine. Additionally, because of SAMe's ability to reduce inflammation and maintain healthy joints, it is being investigated as a possible treatment for osteoarthritis, a degenerative joint condition that affects millions of people globally. Studies exploring its efficacy in treating joint pain and enhancing general joint function have been driven by its role in the creation of proteoglycans, which are essential components of joint cartilage.

HISTORICAL BACKGROUND

When SAMe is examined historically, its journey from a biochemical curiosity to a molecule with significant medicinal potential becomes clear. Its discovery at the beginning of the 1950s was a critical turning point in our comprehension of the complex molecular mechanisms regulating human physiology. Giulio Cantoni's groundbreaking discovery served as a springboard for other investigations that deepened our understanding of the many roles that SAMe plays throughout the body. Researchers, doctors, and consumers have been interested in SAMe for many years, and this has led to several studies and clinical trials looking into its possible health advantages. Its progression from the lab to the world of pharmaceutical therapies and dietary supplements highlights its growing importance in complementary and alternative medicine.

SAMe is still a topic of discussion and research in science as it is investigated for possible uses in a range of medical ailments. Although the exact mechanisms of action and therapeutic efficacy of SAMe have to be determined, its historical development illustrates how it went from being a biochemical curiosity to a potentially useful tool in enhancing general health and well-being. To properly understand its mechanisms of action and demonstrate its usefulness and safety in a variety of therapeutic scenarios, more study is necessary.

CHAPTER TWO

SAME IN HUMAN BODY

THE PART SAME PLAYS

S-adenosyl-L-methionine, or SAMe for short, is an essential substance that is involved in many different bodily metabolic processes. This molecule participates in the transfer of methyl groups to a variety of substrates, such as DNA, proteins, phospholipids, and neurotransmitters, acting as a crucial methyl donor in a myriad of vital events. SAMe plays a complex role in many essential processes, from DNA methylation to neurotransmitter production, which is crucial for preserving general health and well-being.

BIOSYNTHESIS OF SAME

The complex process of one-carbon metabolism, which starts with the transformation of methionine—an important amino acid that can be found in food into SAMe, is the main route by which SAMe production takes place. Methionine adenosyltransferase, an enzyme, is involved in this process. It catalyzes the transfer of the adenosyl group from ATP to methionine, which in turn forms SAMe. This reaction is very sensitive to the amounts of ATP and methionine in cells, which highlights the need for a healthy diet and sufficient nutritional intake for the synthesis of SAMe.

METABOLISM SAME

Apart from its pivotal function in biosynthesis, SAMe metabolism is a strictly regulated process that is crucial for preserving homeostasis in the body. SAMe is transformed into S-adenosylhomocysteine (SAH) by the transfer of the methyl group to an acceptor molecule after it takes part in several methylation processes. Several methyltransferases engaged in a variety of cellular functions support this transition, which ultimately results in the synthesis of SAH, a precursor in the methionine cycle. After that, SAH hydrolyzes to homocysteine, which can either be used in the transsulfuration pathway to synthesize cysteine another essential amino acid or remethylated back to methionine.

Moreover, the metabolism of SAMe is closely associated with the methionine cycle, wherein a complex web of enzymes and co-factors regulates the equilibrium between homocysteine, methionine, and SAMe. Changes in this balance can have a significant impact on several physiological functions, such as the manufacture of neurotransmitters, DNA methylation patterns, and the control of cellular redox balance. Several illnesses, including liver problems, neurodegenerative diseases, and mood disorders, have been linked to imbalances in SAMe metabolism, underscoring the crucial role SAMe plays in preserving general systemic health and functioning.

SAMe plays a variety of vital roles in a range of metabolic pathways within the human body. Its critical function as a methyl donor in many cellular processes highlights how important balanced metabolism and SAMe production are to preserving normal physiological function and general health. Clarifying SAMe's significance in human health and resolving potential imbalances linked to different health disorders requires an understanding of the complexities of its production, metabolism, and role.

CHAPTER THREE

THE ADVANTAGES OF SAME

SAME FOR MENTAL AND MOOD DISORDERS

SAMe, or S-Adenosyl methionine in scientific parlance, is a naturally occurring substance in the human body that is essential to many different metabolic activities. The effects of SAMe on mood and mental health are among the most well-known topics for which it has been thoroughly researched. Scholars have investigated the possible advantages of SAMe in managing mood disorders, including anxiety and depression, in addition to its impact on cognitive abilities.

It's crucial to remember that SAMe contributes to the production of neurotransmitters like dopamine and serotonin, which are directly linked to mood regulation when talking about how SAMe improves mood and mental health. Empirical studies have indicated that SAMe could potentially benefit people with mood disorders by promoting general mental health and emotional stability. This is especially important when discussing depressive illnesses because abnormalities in neurotransmitter levels are frequently seen in these conditions.

DEPRESSION AND SAME

The scientific world has given SAMe's connection to depression a lot of attention. Research has indicated that supplementing with SAMe may be advantageous for people experiencing different types of depression. It is thought that SAMe aids in the synthesis of important neurotransmitters related to mood regulation, which may lessen the symptoms of depression. SAMe is also thought to have a fairly quick start of action, which makes it a viable choice for people who need quick relief from depressive episodes.

Supplementing with SAMe has also been researched about anxiety, another common mental health issue. Although there has been less research on SAMe's direct impact on anxiety than on depression, the initial results point to SAMe's potential involvement in modifying the neurochemical pathways linked to anxiety. Through its effects on neurotransmitter levels and promotion of general brain health, SAMe may help lessen symptoms associated with anxiety. To determine the precise processes and effectiveness of SAMe in treating anxiety disorders, more research is necessary.

COGNITIVE FUNCTION AND SAME

Maintaining cognitive function is essential for preserving general mental health. This includes functions like memory, attention, and reasoning. SAMe may potentially improve cognitive performance, according to certain research findings. Through its facilitation of neurotransmitter synthesis and promotion of optimal brain function, SAMe has the potential to enhance cognitive function and mental acuity in general. To precisely understand the mechanisms behind SAMe's impact on cognitive function and to ascertain its potential involvement in mitigating cognitive loss linked to age and specific neurological disorders, further extensive research is necessary.

Research is now being done on the possible advantages of SAMe for mood and mental health, especially depression and cognitive performance. Even though the amount of research to date is encouraging, further clinical trials are required to determine the effectiveness, ideal dosages, and long-term effects of SAMe.

CHAPTER FOUR

SAME AND WELLNESS

SAME FOR HEALTHY JOINTS

SAMe, also known as S-Adenosyl methionine, is a substance that the body spontaneously produces and is essential to many different metabolic reactions. SAMe has attracted a lot of interest in the field of health and wellness due to its variety of functions, especially when it comes to liver, heart, and joint health.

Supplementing with SAMe has been suggested as a possible way to support joint health, especially for those with osteoarthritis. Joint pain and stiffness are common symptoms of osteoarthritis, a degenerative joint condition marked by the deterioration of joint cartilage and underlying bone. Research indicates that SAMe could facilitate the formation of cartilage and aid in the synthesis of proteoglycans, which could potentially lessen the symptoms of osteoarthritis.

SAMe has demonstrated encouraging anti-inflammatory qualities in the persistent inflammation of joints caused by rheumatoid arthritis, an autoimmune illness. Some studies have suggested that SAMe may help reduce pain and inflammation in people with rheumatoid arthritis, potentially providing a supplementary approach to standard treatment regimens, however further study is needed to firmly confirm its usefulness.

SAME FOR HEPATIC FUNCTION

Moreover, SAMe has demonstrated its importance in preserving liver function. SAMe is necessary for the liver to function at its best because it is an essential organ that is in charge of several metabolic activities. SAMe aids in the production of glutathione, a powerful antioxidant that is essential for liver detoxification. As a result, SAMe has been investigated as a possible treatment for several liver conditions.

SAMe has proven to be able to raise the levels of certain enzymes and raise the liver's general metabolic activity about liver function. SAMe has the potential to be extremely important in maintaining liver function by promoting the synthesis of important chemicals and helping to maintain cellular health, particularly when the liver is subjected to excessive toxins or stressors.

Results with SAMe in the treatment of liver disorders are encouraging. Research has indicated that supplementing with SAMe may be able to slow down the advancement of some liver diseases, including liver cirrhosis and nonalcoholic fatty liver disease (NAFLD). SAMe's anti-inflammatory characteristics and capacity to stimulate liver cell regeneration may help people with a range of liver conditions feel better overall.

HEART HEALTH WITH SAME

Studies on heart health have suggested that SAMe may play a part in improving cardiovascular health. Through its role in homocysteine control, SAMe helps to sustain a healthy cardiovascular system.

Increased risk of cardiovascular illnesses has been linked to elevated homocysteine levels. Because SAMe can control these levels, it may be useful in maintaining heart health and lowering the chance of developing certain cardiovascular diseases.

Additionally, SAMe has been linked to possible advantages in the treatment of hypertension. Initial research has revealed that SAMe may help regulate blood pressure levels, presumably by affecting vascular function and boosting blood flow, but more comprehensive studies are needed to prove its efficacy.

CHAPTER FIVE

SAME AS AN ADD-ON

FORMS AND AMOUNTS

S-adenosyl-l-methionine, or SAMe, is a naturally occurring substance that can be found in nearly all bodily tissues and fluids. Its potential therapeutic effects on a variety of health ailments have made it popular as a supplement, especially when it comes to treating mental disorders, liver conditions, and osteoarthritis. There are several dosages and types of SAMe; choosing the right one for you depends on your demands and other factors.

DISTINCT SAME FORMS

The market offers SAMe in a variety of forms, mostly as tosylate disulfate and butane-disulfonate. Many manufacturers prefer the tosylate disulfate version because it is more stable and has a longer shelf life. However, it is thought that the butane-disulfonate form is more susceptible to temperature changes and humidity, which could have an impact on its stability. Nonetheless, both versions have proven effective in numerous clinical trials, and the decision between the two typically boils down to the user's particular needs and preferences.

CHOOSING THE APPROPRIATE DOSAGE

To achieve the intended therapeutic effects without suffering from negative side effects, figuring out the appropriate dosage of SAMe is essential. Depending on the illness being treated, the person's general health, and any additional medications or supplements being used, there may be differences in the right dosage. Seeking advice from a healthcare expert who can take these things into account and offer tailored advice is advised. Initial doses for osteoarthritis typically lie between 600 and 1200 mg/day, and doses for mood support may vary from 400 to

1600 mg/day. Individual reactions, however, could differ, and depending on the user's unique health profile, dose modifications might be required.

SELECTING THE APPROPRIATE SAME SUPPLEMENT

Selecting the best SAMe supplement requires taking into account several important criteria. First and foremost, you must choose a manufacturer who is respected, trustworthy, and has a track record of upholding stringent quality control requirements. It's also important to understand the supplement's potency and purity because some products could have extra components or fillers that reduce their efficiency or have unintended adverse effects. Furthermore, it's crucial to look at the supplement's form—enteric-coated or not—because the former may help some people avoid gastrointestinal adverse effects.

ASPECTS TO THINK ABOUT

When choosing a SAMe supplement, factors to take into account are the product's bioavailability, affordability, and the existence of extra regulatory authority certifications, like the U.S. The NSF International or the USP Pharmacopeia. These certifications give customers additional peace of mind regarding the safety and effectiveness of the product by guaranteeing that the supplement has undergone stringent testing for quality and purity.

CHAPTER SIX

POSSIBLE ADVERSE REACTIONS AND CONCURRENT EVENTS

FREQUENT ADVERSE EVENTS

The expected negative reactions to a specific drug or treatment that usually affect a large proportion of patients are known as common side effects. Depending on the particular drug, its mode of action, and the patient's particular reaction to the treatment, these effects can differ greatly. The most commonly reported adverse effects include headaches, nausea, exhaustion, dizziness, and constipation. Other typical side effects include gastrointestinal disturbances including diarrhea and constipation, as well as moderate allergic reactions such as skin rashes or itching. Even though these adverse effects are typically minor and self-limiting, they can nevertheless have a major negative effect on a patient's quality of life and may require changing the dosage or course of treatment.

Common adverse effects occasionally become dose-dependent, which means that when the medicine is taken at higher dosages, the negative effects happen more frequently or more strongly. To ensure that patients are receiving the most effective dosage while limiting the possibility of experiencing unwanted effects, this calls for close monitoring by healthcare professionals. Additionally, patient education regarding typical side effects is essential to foster comprehension and control expectations, empowering people to choose their treatments wisely and know when to seek medical attention.

DRUG-DRUG RELATIONS

Drug interactions happen when the presence of another substance, whether it be food, drink, or another medication, alters the effects of the first medication. This can lead to unexpected changes in the toxicity, efficacy, or pharmacological action of one or both substances. These interactions may have several negative impacts, such as decreased therapeutic efficacy, an increased chance of side effects, or the emergence of potentially dangerous substances within the body. Drug interactions can take many different forms, including changes in the medications' distribution, excretion, metabolism, absorption, or overall effectiveness. These changes can have a significant effect on the treatments' overall safety and effectiveness.

An essential part of safe and efficient medication management is comprehending and controlling drug interactions. To evaluate the possibility of interactions, healthcare professionals need to consider a patient's whole medication profile, which includes prescription, over-the-counter, and dietary supplements. To avoid the possibility of harmful drug interactions, individuals should also be urged to tell their healthcare professionals about all substances they are currently taking. To reduce the risk of dangerous medication combinations, pharmacists and other healthcare professionals are essential in spotting possible interactions and giving prescribers and patients the advice they need. Furthermore, pharmacogenomics has made it possible to take a more individualized approach to treatment by taking into account a person's genetic composition when predicting how they will react to specific drugs and any potential interactions.

CHAPTER SEVEN

PARTICULAR POPULATIONS AND SAME

SAME YOUNGSTERS

SAMe, also known as S-Adenosyl methionine, is a well-liked dietary supplement that supports several physiological processes. It has drawn interest due to its possible health advantages. However, using it on minors needs to be done with caution and under close supervision. Although SAMe is created by the body naturally and is safe for adults in proper amounts, there is still a dearth of research on its use in pediatric populations. There is a paucity of clinical data regarding the use of SAMe in children, thus caution should be exercised when considering its administration in this population.

The possible effects of SAMe use on children's developing physiological systems are among the main worries. Children's metabolic pathways are complex, and their body composition and weight vary widely, therefore it's important to fully comprehend how SAMe affects these sensitive systems. In addition, it is important to thoroughly investigate how SAMe can interact with other drugs or supplements that are frequently prescribed for kids to avoid any negative side effects or unexpected outcomes.

SAME FOR SENIOR CITIZENS

Elderly people frequently struggle with a variety of health issues, such as mood disorders, joint health, and cognitive function. As an additional therapeutic, SAMe has demonstrated encouraging promise. Research findings suggest that SAMe may contribute to maintaining joint health by facilitating the synthesis of proteoglycans, which are vital constituents of joint cartilage. Furthermore, because it is involved in the manufacture of neurotransmitters such as norepinephrine, dopamine, and serotonin, research has been conducted into its potential effects on mood regulation. This is important because mood disorders like anxiety and depression are frequently seen in the elderly.

However, there are several things to keep in mind when using SAMe in older adults. When providing SAMe, careful monitoring is required due to many factors, including age-related changes in metabolism, concurrent pharmaceutical use, and the presence of underlying medical problems. Furthermore, the possibility of interactions between SAMe and routinely prescribed drugs for the elderly highlights the significance of healthcare practitioners being aware of SAMe's use in this demographic.

SAME THROUGHOUT HER PREGNANCY AND NURSING

The health and welfare of the developing fetus and the mother are of utmost importance during pregnancy and lactation. Although SAMe is an essential component of many physiological processes and is found naturally in the body, its use during pregnancy and lactation should be carefully considered because there isn't much information on its safety and effectiveness in these particular populations. Concerns about SAMe's possible impacts on prenatal development and the health of the infant highlight the need for caution when thinking about supplementing during these crucial times.

Additionally, worries regarding SAMe's effects on the nursing newborn are raised by the possibility that it will be transferred through breast milk. It is recommended that nursing moms speak with their healthcare professionals before starting SAMe on their regimen due to the incomplete knowledge of the drug's effects on newborn development and possible interactions with the infant's metabolic processes.

CHAPTER EIGHT

INCLUDING SAME IN YOUR DAILY ACTIVITIES

DIET AND SAME

S-adenosyl-methionine, or SAMe, is a substance that the human body naturally contains and is essential to many different metabolic activities. It has a role in the synthesis of neurotransmitters, the construction of cell membranes, and mood control. Including SAMe in your diet can have several positive effects on your health, especially when it comes to joint and mental health. In addition to food sources, a balanced diet and nutritional supplements can help sustain SAMe and promote a healthy lifestyle in general.

SOURCES OF SAME IN DIET

SAMe can be acquired from the diet, however not in large quantities in many foods. Its main source is methionine, an important amino acid that can be found in a variety of foods high in protein, including dairy, meat, and fish. In addition, the body can generate SAMe by methylating methionine, a process that needs sufficient nutrition, including magnesium, folate, and the vitamins B6 and B12. Consequently, eating a diet high in these nutrients can help the body produce SAMe naturally in an indirect way.

SAME AND DIETARY ASSISTANCE

When it comes to nutritional support, a common way to incorporate SAMe into your lifestyle is to think about taking supplements that offer a synthetic version of this chemical. SAMe pills or capsules are a popular form of these supplements. Usually, they are employed to lessen the symptoms of illnesses including depression, osteoarthritis, and liver problems. It is crucial to speak with a healthcare provider before pursuing nutritional support through SAMe supplements to establish the right dosage and make sure it won't conflict with any current prescriptions or medical issues.

Including foods high in vitamins and minerals that are known to stimulate the formation of SAMe in your diet will further enhance the advantages of introducing SAMe into your lifestyle. Consuming foods high in folate, such as citrus fruits, legumes, and leafy green vegetables, is essential for promoting the body's production of SAMe.

Furthermore, eating foods strong in vitamin B12, like dairy, fish, and meat, can aid in the production of

SAMe. Additionally, consuming whole grains, nuts, and seeds high in magnesium and vitamin B6 can aid in the body's natural synthesis of SAMe.

In general, those who want to maximize their physical and mental well-being must comprehend the connection between SAMe and nutrition.

While there are certain dietary sources of SAMe, to address particular health conditions, it may be helpful to provide nutritional support through supplements. People might potentially improve their general health and well-being by consuming a well-rounded diet that includes nutrients that encourage the creation of SAMe. This is because people will benefit from the benefits of this key molecule for numerous bodily functions.

CHAPTER NINE

SAME IN COMBINATION WITH OTHER SUPPLEMENTS

COOPERATION WITH OTHER ELEMENTS

SAMe, or S-adenosyl-L-methionine, is a naturally occurring substance that can be found in nearly all bodily tissues and fluids. It is essential for several metabolic processes, such as the creation of neurotransmitters, the methylation of DNA, and the upkeep of cell membranes. SAMe's overall therapeutic potential can be increased when it is paired with specific additional nutrients to provide synergistic benefits. An instance of this can be observed in its interplay with certain nutrients, specifically B vitamins, specifically B12 and folic acid, which play a role in the methylation process. Together with these vitamins, SAMe promotes healthy nervous system operation and mood management.

VITAMIN SUPPLEMENTS AND SAME

When it comes to dietary supplements, SAMe and multivitamins together can offer complete support for general health. A range of vital nutrients, including vitamins A, C, D, E, and several B vitamins, are frequently found in multivitamins.

These nutrients support the function of SAMe in preserving proper physiological functioning. Together, they can help with immunological support, energy production, and mood management, among other aspects of health. Since taking too much of some nutrients can have negative consequences, it's crucial to make sure the multivitamin and SAMe dosages are within acceptable bounds and don't go over the daily allotment.

SUGGESTIONS FOR SAME SUPPLEMENTATION THAT WORKS

It's critical to take into account a few crucial elements to optimize the advantages of SAMe supplementation.

First and foremost, you must speak with a healthcare provider before starting SAMe, particularly if you have any underlying medical issues or are taking other drugs. Second, lowering the dose initially and progressively raising it as directed by a medical professional can lessen the possibility of negative effects. Furthermore, consuming SAMe with a light meal or empty stomach can improve its absorption, guaranteeing its effectiveness. To preserve its stability, SAMe should also be kept out of direct sunlight and in a cold, dry location.

Following recommended procedures is essential when using SAMe with other supplements to guarantee the greatest possible health results. A stable blood level of SAMe can be maintained by creating and following a dose regimen, which will support the drug's long-lasting therapeutic benefits. To avoid any negative responses, it's also critical to be aware of any possible interactions between SAMe and other supplements or drugs. Getting advice from a healthcare professional can help you make sense of the intricate relationships between supplements and create a customized supplementation strategy that fits your needs.

OBSERVING AND MODIFYING

It is essential to regularly observe how the body reacts to SAMe supplementation to evaluate its safety and effectiveness. This means keeping an eye out for any shifts in mood, energy, and general well-being, as well as any possible negative consequences. Depending on the patient's reaction and any changes in their health, the dosage or regimen may need to be adjusted. Consulting a healthcare professional regularly can help ensure that SAMe supplementation is optimized and continues to be a safe and beneficial part of an all-encompassing wellness plan.

CHAPTER TEN

THE PROSPECTS FOR SAME STUDIES

CURRENT RESEARCH AND UPCOMING PROJECTS

Research on SAMe's ongoing applications and future directions is primarily concerned with comprehending the complex mechanisms underlying its action and investigating its possible applications in a range of therapeutic domains. SAMe, also known as S-Adenosyl methionine, is a substance that the body spontaneously produces and is essential to many different metabolic reactions. Its many functions and potential advantages have been the subject of intense research, opening the door to many fascinating developments in the healthcare and medical industries.

RECENT RESEARCH

A noteworthy feature of the field of SAMe research is the investigation of its impact on mental health. Recent research has indicated that there may be a connection between taking supplements high in SAMe and treating mental health issues like anxiety and depression. By learning more about the neurochemical pathways that SAMe may use to regulate mood, researchers hope to shed light on the intricate relationship that exists between biochemical processes and emotional health.

Moreover, continuing research initiatives are also concentrating their attention on SAMe's significance in alleviating the negative impacts of liver disorders. Hepatic illnesses, particularly liver cirrhosis and nonalcoholic fatty liver disease (NAFLD), have been of special attention, considering SAMe's significance in supporting liver function and facilitating detoxification processes. Researchers are investigating the potential of SAMe supplementation in ameliorating liver damage, thereby offering promising prospects for the development of novel therapeutic interventions targeting liver-related ailments.

Furthermore, the exploration of SAMe's impact on joint health and its potential in managing conditions such as osteoarthritis has garnered substantial attention. As musculoskeletal disorders continue to pose a significant burden on global healthcare systems, the investigation of SAMe's role in supporting joint function and alleviating inflammation has become a crucial area of interest. Researchers are actively conducting clinical trials and preclinical studies to elucidate the underlying mechanisms and assess the efficacy of SAMe in improving joint mobility and reducing discomfort associated with degenerative joint diseases.

POTENTIAL APPLICATIONS

In addition to its role in mental health, liver function, and joint health, emerging studies are also indicating the potential applications of SAMe in addressing neurodegenerative diseases. Researchers are exploring the neuroprotective effects of SAMe, considering its capacity to modulate neurotransmitter levels and enhance neuronal function. With the prevalence of neurodegenerative disorders such as Alzheimer's and Parkinson's diseases, the investigation of SAMe's neuroprotective properties represents a promising avenue for the development of innovative therapeutic strategies aimed at mitigating cognitive decline and preserving brain health.

Overall, the future of SAMe research appears promising, with ongoing studies and emerging findings underscoring its potential applications across various domains, including mental health, liver function, joint health, and neuroprotection. As researchers continue to unravel the intricate mechanisms underlying SAMe's biological actions, the insights garnered from these investigations are poised to pave the way for the development of novel treatment modalities and the enhancement of healthcare practices, ultimately contributing to the advancement of human well-being and quality of life.

CHAPTER ELEVEN

CHALLENGES FACED

In the realm of modern healthcare, an array of challenges constantly confronts healthcare professionals, necessitating adaptive strategies and dynamic solutions. These challenges arise from multifaceted sources, ranging from the complexities of technological advancements and rapidly evolving treatment modalities to the intricacies of patient care and resource management. One of the foremost predicaments pertains to the intricate balance between providing quality patient care and managing the ever-increasing administrative burden, which often encumbers the precious time and resources of healthcare professionals. The ever-evolving regulatory landscape and compliance requirements further compound these challenges, often demanding meticulous attention to detail and adherence to stringent protocols, which can impede the efficiency of healthcare delivery.

Furthermore, the perpetual issue of limited resources, including funding, staffing, and infrastructure, poses a persistent obstacle in the pursuit of optimal healthcare provision. In the face of burgeoning patient populations, escalating healthcare costs, and disparities in access to care, healthcare professionals often find themselves stretched thin, struggling to meet the demands of an increasingly complex and diverse patient demographic. The scarcity of specialized expertise and the need for continuous professional development add additional layers of complexity, necessitating a dynamic approach to knowledge acquisition and skill enhancement within the healthcare workforce.

In addition to these systemic challenges, healthcare professionals also grapple with the emotional toll of providing care in high-pressure environments. Witnessing human suffering, coping with patient loss, and navigating complex ethical dilemmas can profoundly impact the mental and emotional well-being of healthcare professionals. Burnout, compassion fatigue, and moral distress are just a few manifestations of the psychological strain experienced by healthcare professionals, which not only affect individual well-being but also have implications for patient care and overall healthcare outcomes.

HEALTHCARE PROFESSIONALS' PERSPECTIVES

From the healthcare professionals' perspective, these challenges underscore the need for comprehensive support systems, including robust institutional frameworks, effective interdisciplinary collaboration, and prioritization of mental health and well-being initiatives. Creating an environment that fosters open communication, promotes a culture of empathy and understanding, and advocates for work-life balance is essential in addressing the multifaceted challenges faced by healthcare professionals. Embracing technological innovations that streamline administrative tasks, enhance patient engagement, and facilitate evidence-based decision-making can also alleviate the burden on healthcare professionals, enabling them to focus more effectively on patient care and holistic well-being.

Ultimately, by acknowledging and addressing the challenges faced by healthcare professionals, stakeholders within the healthcare ecosystem can work collaboratively towards fostering a resilient and sustainable healthcare infrastructure that not only prioritizes patient outcomes but also recognizes and supports the invaluable contributions of the healthcare workforce.

www.ingramcontent.com/pod-product-compliance
Lightning Source LLC
Chambersburg PA
CBHW060757260726
48660CB00002B/669